I0759356

My Sistah's Pantry

FEATURING: MY MEDICINE CABINET

WRITTEN BY:

PROFESSOR KELMER ELIZABETH MUHAMMAD

Introduction

NOTE: It is always best to consult with a physician or a naturopathic doctor before changing your diet regiment.

"My Medicine Cabinet" is a modest homeopathic book that provides simple herbs and spices, and home remedies to store in your kitchen cabinet or your pantry. This book provides basic ingredients that will aid in digestion, boost the immune system, aide in inflammation, weight loss, and much more. Rather than buy all the herbs and spices in the market place, "My Medicine Cabinet" provides basic ingredients and recipes that are easily obtainable, easily stored, and easy to make. The homeopathic remedies and ingredients listed in this book is a prescription to preventative medicine.

How to Store Foods

Canning or pickling foods can last up to 5 to 10 years. Invest in glass jars (i.e. mason jars). Foods that are canned in tin, run the risk of botulism. Most commercial food cans are lined with a chemical called, "epoxy resin." Epoxy resin contains bisphenol A (BPA) which is a chemical used to make plastics. The Food and Drug Administration (FDA) states that BPA is safe to consume at low levels.

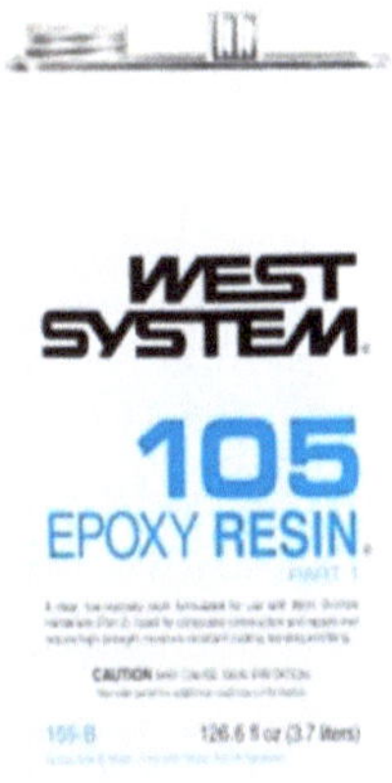

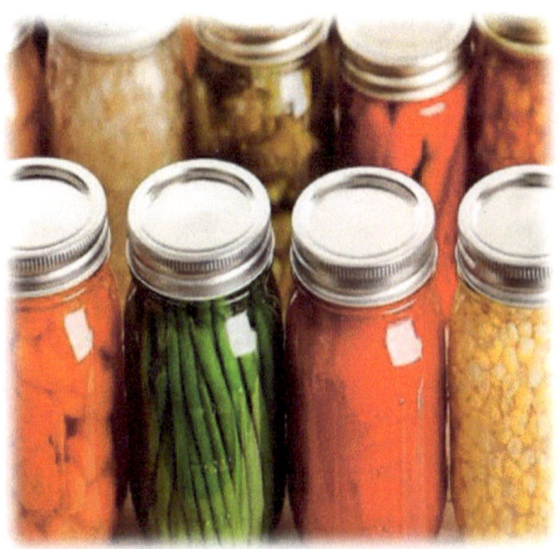

Simple Foods

You do not have to eat everything that people say is good to eat.

According to Mr. Elijah Muhammad, "You do not need everything that is good to eat to live a happy life. Take some of the things that are good to eat. Of course, you should have a balanced diet (How to Eat to Live Book One)." Too much food and too many different types of food for our body to digest efficiently will make you tired after eating a simple meal. Simple foods are easier to obtain, easily digestible, and will make your body feel better.

The Navy Bean

The most important food to store in your food pantry is the navy bean. The navy bean (small white bean) is considered one of the healthiest beans on the market. It got its name from the United States Navy in the early 20th Century. The Navy bean has several beneficial factors: it's a rich source of dietary fiber; loaded in protein; low in fat; highly rich in iron; regulates metabolism; and is good for the skin. If you eat this bean every day, it will provide all nutrients and supplements needed to abstain life.

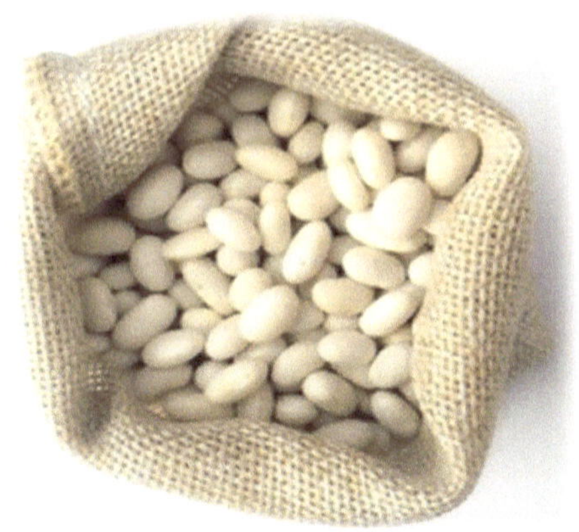
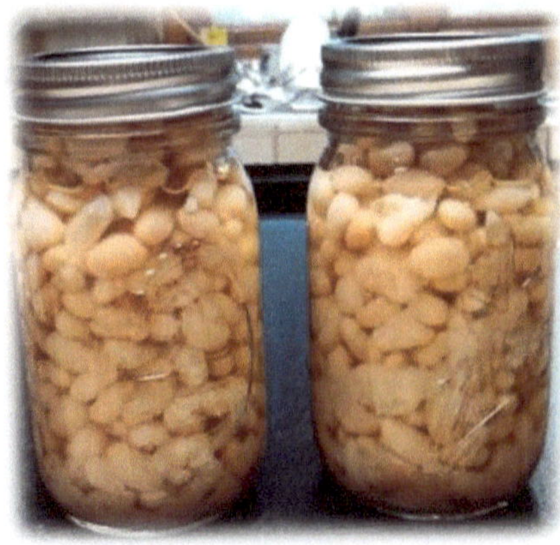

Basic Navy Bean Soup

1. Soak Beans over night or place clean washed beans in a pressure cooker
2. 1 Quart of Water to a Bag of Beans. Boil to Soft.
3. 1 Pint of Vegetable or Chicken Stock
4. ½ Cup vegetables – Garlic, Onion, Carrots, red and green peppers (sautéed in 1 tablespoon of olive oil)
5. 1 Teaspoon Seasonings paprika, onion, garlic, thyme, oregano, and turmeric
6. 1 can Tomato Paste or Tomato Sauce (Optional)
7. Add Kosher Salt last to taste.

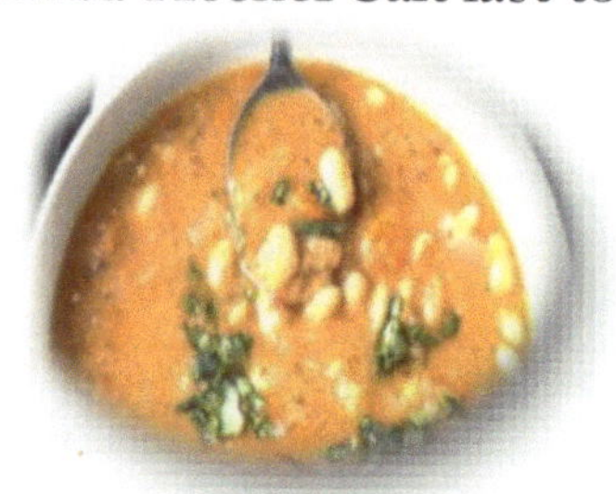

Add vegetable stock to soft beans. Sautéed vegetables in 1 tablespoon of Olive Oil in a saucepan. Add to soft beans. Mix in tomatoes if you want it red. Add seasonings and salt; then simmer. If you have a pressure cooker, place all ingredients into the pot, set the timer and let cook for approximately 15 to 20 minutes (wash beans and pick out any rocks before cooking). Personally, I recommend to soak beans for over night to void intestinal gas.

Lentil Beans

Lentils are small legumes (beans) that are high in fiber and nutrients. This bean packs about 25% protein that can be substituted for meat. Also, it is a great source of iron and an excellent source of B vitamins. These beans are inexpensive to store and can provide nutrients to abstain a healthy life.

Lentile Bean Soup

1 ½ cups green lentils

1 zucchini squash, diced

2 celery stalks, chopped

Salt and pepper

1 tsp ground cumin

½ tsp ground cinnamon

3 cups canned diced tomatoes

Olive Oil

1 bulk carrot, diced

1 russet potato, diced

1 tsp ground coriander

1 tsp turmeric powder

½ tsp cayenne pepper

2 ½ cup water

1 cup chopped fresh parsley, stems removed

Soak beans for 15 minutes. Sautee' vegetables in olive oil. Add tomatoes, seasonings and vegetables to lentils and cook over medium heat.

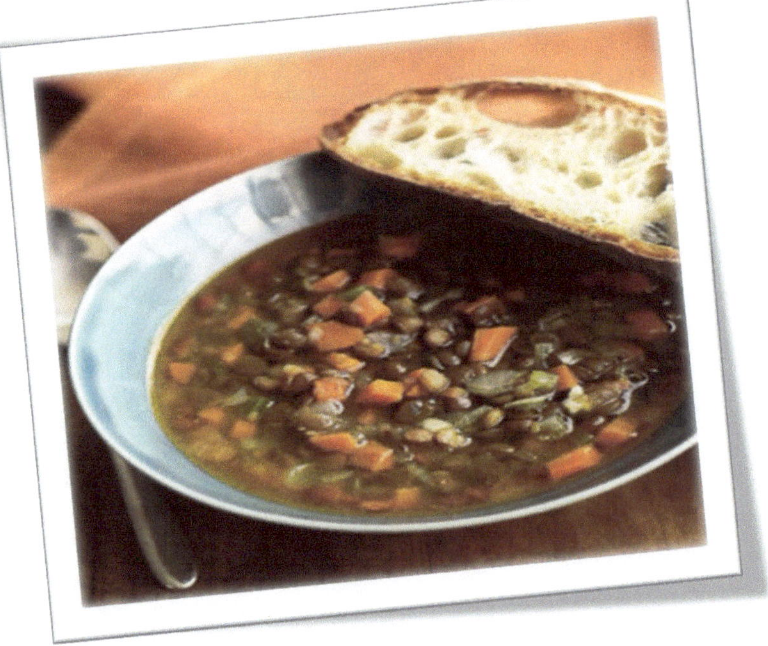

Flours, Grains, & Rice

Flours, grains, and rice are great to have in your pantry. They are a great investment because they can fill up the belly. Unfortunately, these food items should be stored in the refrigerator or freezer for at least 3 to 5 days in order to kill those pesky little bugs called, "Wheat Weevils." Weevils usually infest grains and starches like rice, flour, pasta, and cereals; fortunately, they are not dangerous. To void an outbreak or an infestation place flour in food grade containers and place in the freezer for at least 2 days; this will destroy the larvae (eggs) that lay dormant in the flour for approximately five months.

Wheat & Unbleached Flours

Wheat Flour

Wheat flour produces gluten, a protein that imparts strength and elasticity to dough; it influences the texture of baked goods. Most flour is a mixture of hard and soft wheat.

Unbleached Flour

Do not buy bleached flour. It is treated with chemical agents to speed up the aging process. Unbleached flour is highly recommended; it has aged naturally after being milled. Finally, unbleached flour is light and used to bake breads, cakes, and crusts.

Oatmeal, Malto-Meal & Cream of Wheat

Oatmeal, Malto-Meal, and Cream of Wheat are farinas (milled wheat) that is great for cooking and helps to regulate digestion. Farinas are excellent storage grains and great fillers to start the day.

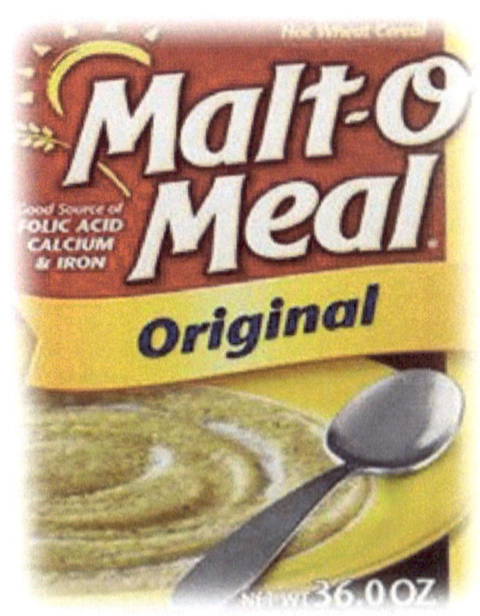

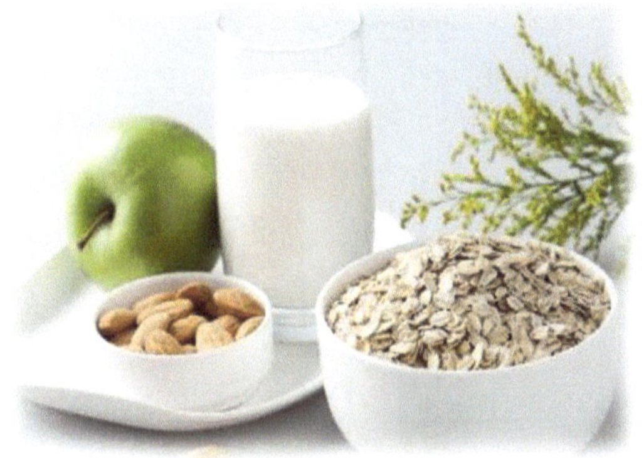

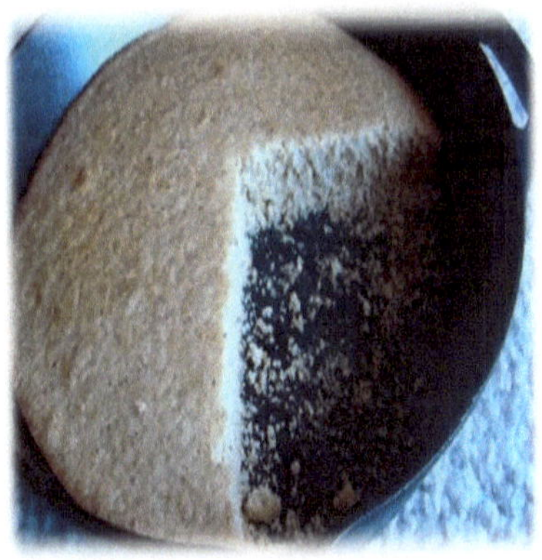

Brown Rice

If it floats at the bottom, it's rice; if it floats on top, it's plastic!

Eating a bowl of rice may make your gut happy. The fiber in rice may play a role in obtaining a healthy diet. The best rice to store is the brown rice. If you have white rice such as Basmati, wash it and bake it in the oven until its brown. Also store your rice in the freezer to void Wheat Weevils.

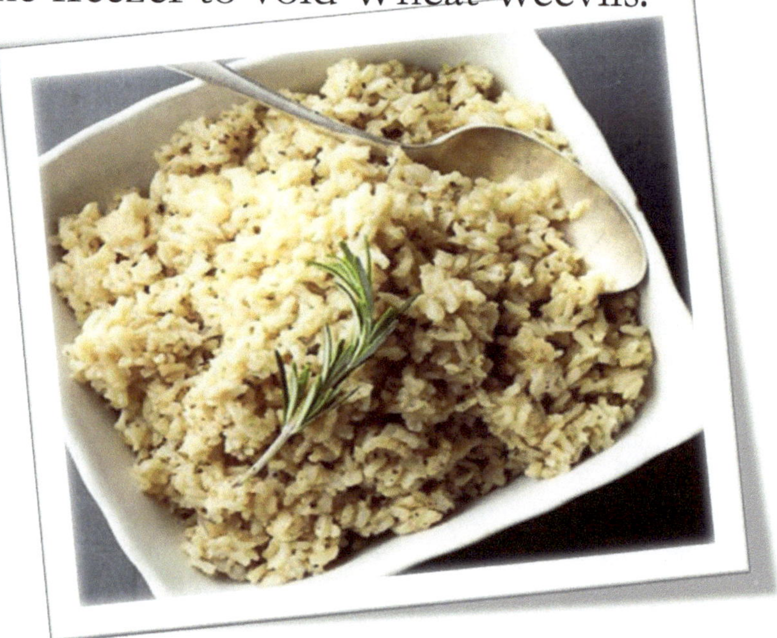

9 Healthy Fats & Oils

Saturated and Mono-unsaturated fats are healthy choices to cook with. They are also good for the skin, hair, and body.

NOTE: AVOID COOKING WITH PEANUT, CORN, CANOLA, AND SOYBEAN OILS; ALSO, ANIMAL FATS (ESPECIALLY LARD)!

1. Olive Oil
2. Avocado Oil
3. Sunflower Oil
4. Butter and/or Ghee
5. Grapeseed Oil
6. Coconut Oil
7. Flaxseed Oil
8. Raw Cacao Butter
9. **Blackseed Oil

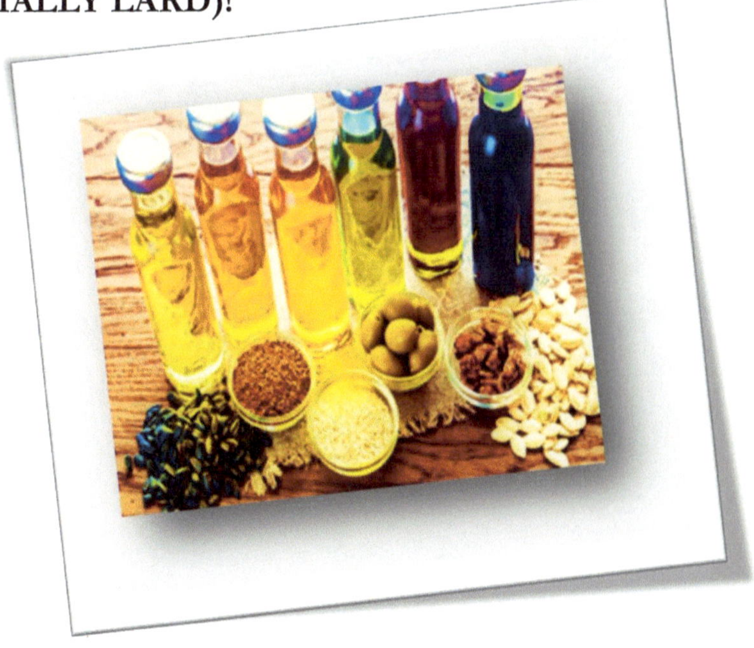

Blackseed Oil

Most people are not aware of the properties and benefits of blackseed oil. Black seed oil is extracted from the seeds of black cumin. It can boost the immune system, reduce inflammation, and fight infections. Although this oil is good to have on hand, taking too much may harm your liver and kidneys.

19 Herbs & Spices to Store in Your Medicine Cabinet

Forget about Colonel Sanders' 11 herbs and spices; store these 19 ingredients to flavor foods and beverages!

1. Allspice
2. Anise
3. Bay Leaves
4. Basil
5. Cayenne Pepper
6. Chili Peppers
7. Cinnamon
8. Cloves
9. Dried Mustard
10. Ginger
11. Kosher Salt
12. Marjoram
13. Onion
14. Oregano
15. Paprika
16. Peppercorns
17. Sage
18. Thyme
19. Turmeric

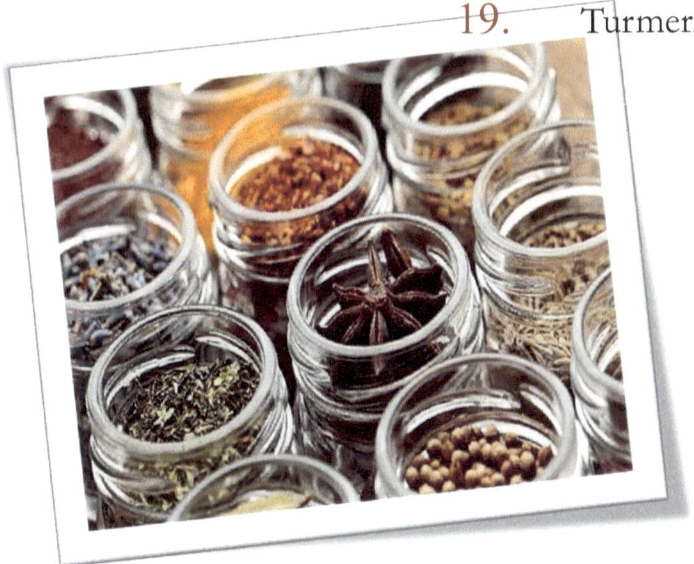

9 Simple Metabolism & Immune Boosters

There are plenty of foods that can boost your immune system; however, if you are on a low budget, these simple ingredients are inexpensive, easily obtainable, and can be made into elixirs, teas, and fermented (for medicinal purpose).

1. Citrus Fruits
2. Dark Chocolate - Cacao
3. Garlic
4. Ginger
5. Onion
6. Raw Apple Cider Vinegar
7. Raw Honey
8. Turmeric
9. Hot Peppers

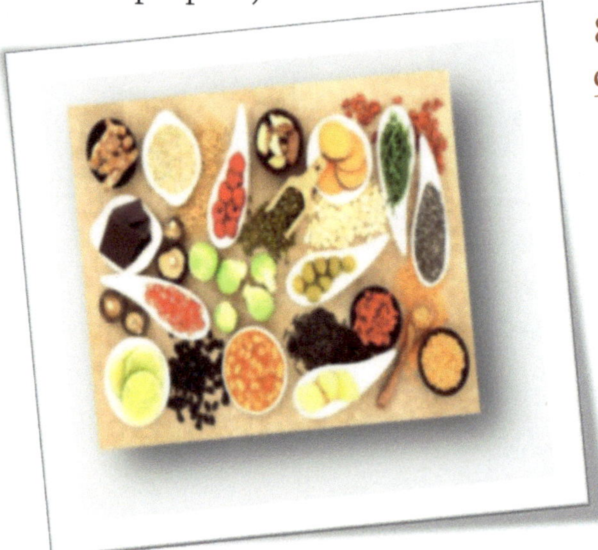

Benefits & Properties of 9 Simple Foods

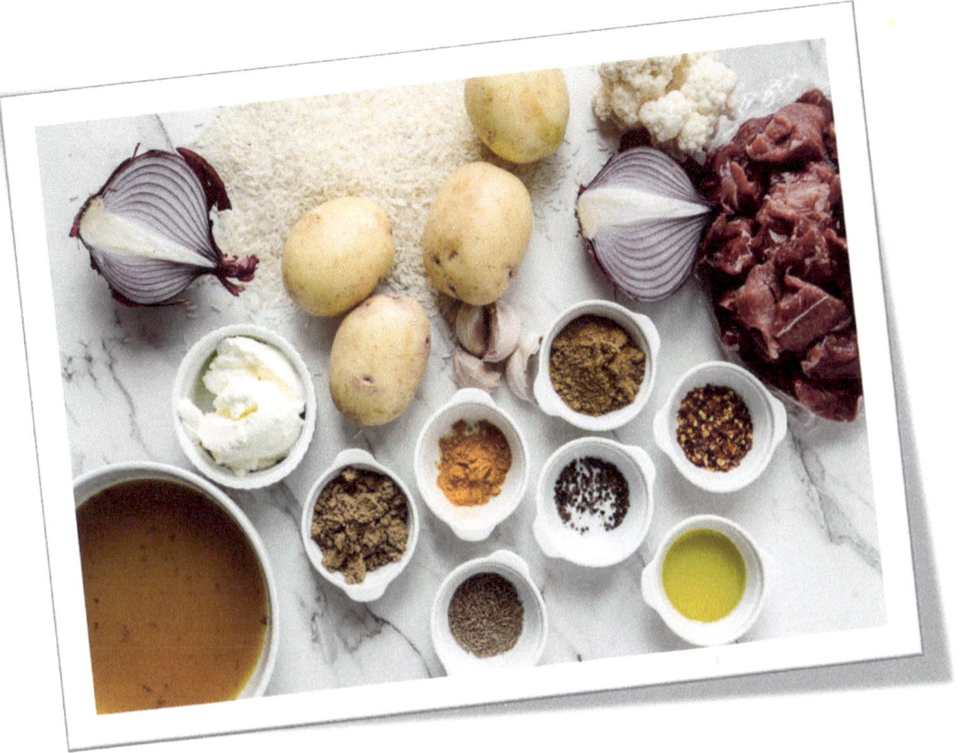

1. Citrus Fruits

Citrus Fruits is an excellent source of immune-boosting vitamin C. Oranges, lemons, limes, tangerines, and grapefruits are packed with nutrients and flavors that makes a great addition to a healthy diet. There are Five amazing benefits of eating citrus fruits.

- Good for the heart
- Low glycemic index (will not spike your blood sugar)
- They are hydrating
- Weight loss Staple
- Good Source of Fiber

2. Dark Chocolate or Cacao

Raw organic cacao has over 40 times the antioxidants of blueberries. Normal cocoa powder and chocolate have been chemically processed and roasted, which destroys antioxidants and flavanols (the things that keep you young and healthy). Cacao is one of the highest plant-based sources of iron. It is a great source of an immune booster.

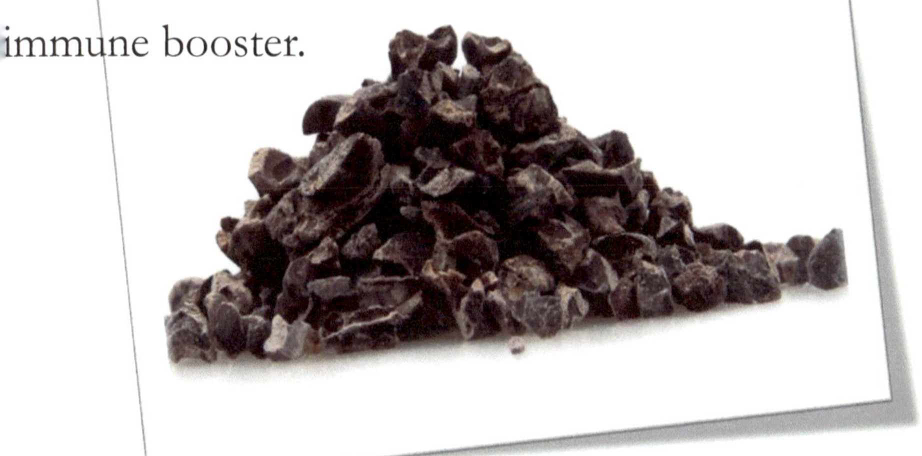

3. Garlic

Garlic is an herb that is grown around the world and easily obtainable. It produces a chemical called allicin, which causes garlic to smell. Garlic is used for many conditions related to the heart and blood system (i.e. high blood pressure and atherosclerosis). There are five uses and benefits that are great for the immune system.

1. Diabetes
2. Control High Cholesterol
3. Prostate Cancer
4. Aid in tick bites
5. Aid in Ringworms

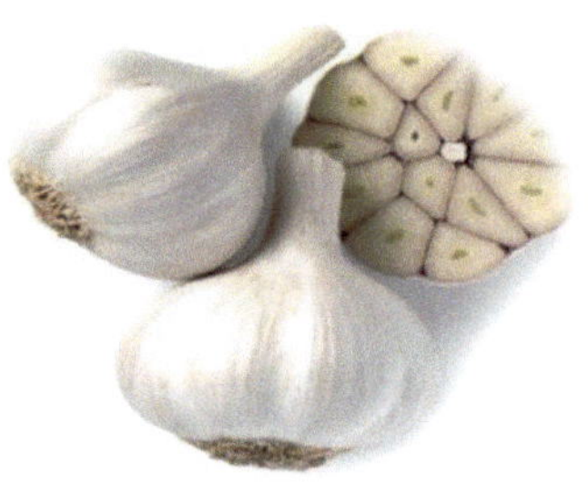

Garlic Soup

This recipe will help to fight off the flu and colds

- 1 tablespoon olive oil
- 12 cloves fresh peeled garlic
- 2 large, sweet yellow onions,
- 1 teaspoon fresh thyme
- 1 cup chicken broth or vegetable bouillon
- 1 cup of cream
- 1 pinch cayenne pepper, or more to taste
- 1 tablespoon fresh basil, chopped and Salt

On low heat, sauté the garlic and onions in a saucepan and covered for about 25 minutes until cooked through. Transfer the garlic and onions to a food processor or blender and puree with the thyme and 1/2 cup of the broth or bouillon. Pour the puree back into the pan, add the remaining broth, and simmer for 20 minutes. Stir in the cayenne, basil, and salt to taste, and heat for 2 minutes.

4. Ginger

Ginger is one of the healthiest spices on earth. The rhizome is the part that is commonly used as a spice. It is called the ginger root or ginger. Ginger can be used fresh, dried, powdered or as an oil. Here are three great health benefits:

1. Ginger has long been used for culinary and medicinal purpose.

2. Possible health benefits include reducing nausea, pain, and inflammation.

3. Chewing raw ginger or drinking ginger tea is a common home remedy for nausea during cancer treatment.

5. Onions

Onions are part of the allium family of vegetables and herbs, which also includes chives, garlic, scallions, and leeks. They have antihistamine effects due to quercetin, an antioxidant that acts like an antihistamine and an anti-inflammatory. The most common types are red, yellow, and white onions.

- Decreases the risk of overall mortality, diabetes, and heart disease.
- Promotes a healthful complexion, hair, increased energy, and overall lower weight.
- Lowers the risk of colon, prostate, and stomach cancers
- Folate, which is found in onions, helps to reduce depression

6. Raw Apple Cider Vinegar – ACV

Six Benefits of Apple Cider Vinegar

1. Can Kill Types of Harmful Bacteria such as E. Coli

2. Lower Blood Sugar Levels and Fights Diabetes

3. Helps to Lose Weight and Reduces Body Fat

4. Lowers Cholesterol and Helps to Improves a Healthy Heart

5. Protective Effects Against Cancer Agents

6. Can be used to Clean your Fruits and Vegetables

The main component in apple cider vinegar is acetic acid. In addition, it contains substances such as lactic, citric, malic acids and bacteria. ACV contains about three calories per tablespoon, which is very low. Also, it can be used for other non-health related uses such as hair conditioning, skin care, dental care, pet use and as a cleaning agent.

How to Make Apple Cider Vinegar

- 5 to 10 apples of your choice
- 2 quarts mason jar
- Tablespoon of raw sugar to every apple or raw honey
- 4 to 6 cups of water

Cut apples including core, seeds, and stem and place in a mason jar. Add sugar to water and stir with a wooden spoon (**do not use any type of metal spoon**). Pour sugar water into mason jar. Make sure every apple is immersed in the water solution. Place a cover on top of the jar. You can use a coffee filter with a rubber ban or a simple lid. Set the jar aside and open the lid every 2 or 3 days to release gases for at least 2 to 3 weeks. Don't worry about seeing bubbles. The chemical reaction is acid and bacteria, which is are natural responses. Let jar sit on the counter for approximately a month. Finally, after a month, strain the apples with a cheese cloth, drink and refrigerate!

7. Raw Honey

Honey that are on shelves of grocery stores is pasteurized. In fact, many of the beneficial nutrients are destroyed because of the use of high heat that is destroyed in the process. Raw honey or unfiltered can be found at local farmer's market or honey hive farms. The great thing about honey, it never spoils and can be stored for years. Here are five great benefits of raw honey:

1. A good source of antioxidants

2. Antibacterial and antifungal properties

3. Heal wounds

4. Help for digestive issues

5. Helps Improve Cholesterol

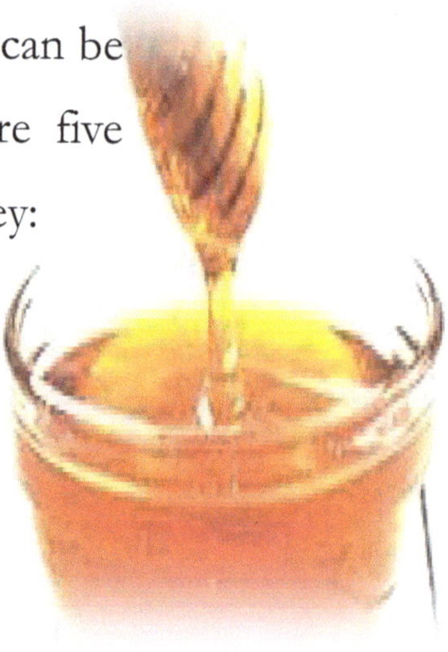

8. Turmeric

Turmeric is the spice that gives curry its yellow color. It has anti-inflammatory effects and a strong antioxidant. It also helps your body fight foreign invaders and has a role in repairing damage.

1. Boost Immunity
2. Treats Asthma
3. Anti-Inflammatory Agent
4. Strong Anti-Oxidant
5. Boost Digestion

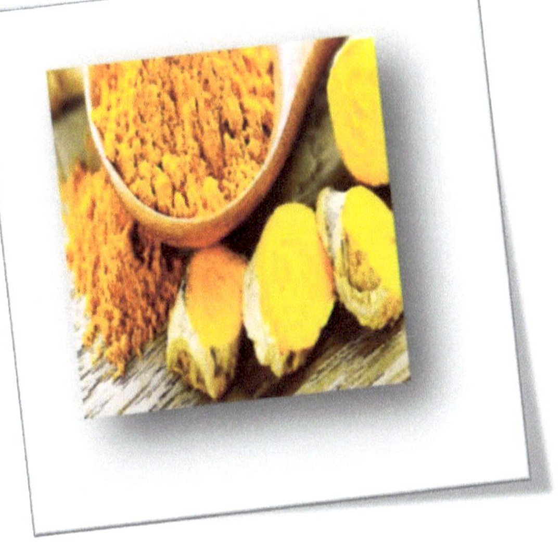

9. Hot Peppers

Adding hot peppers or hot powders to food continues to protect us from food poisoning. Capsaicin's anti-microbial properties, which is the main ingredient in all hot peppers inhibit as much as 75% of bacteria growth. The following is a list of health benefits of eating hot peppers:

1. Aids in the Circulatory System
2. Helps to Relieve Migraines
3. Applied to the Skin to Relieve Joint Pains
4. Improves Metabolism and Weight Loss
5. Fights Flus, Colds and Fungal Infections

Additional Foods for Storage

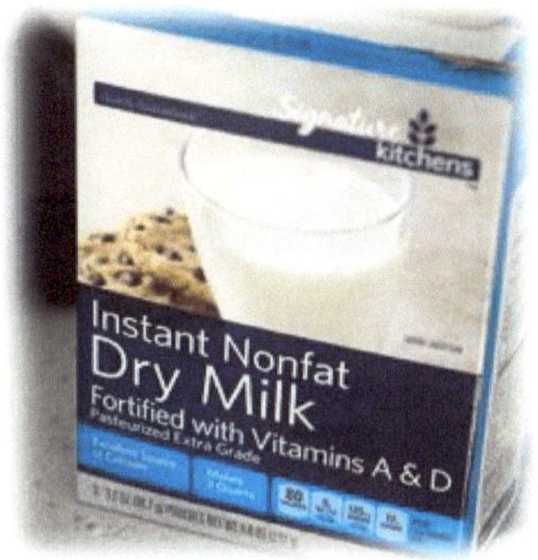

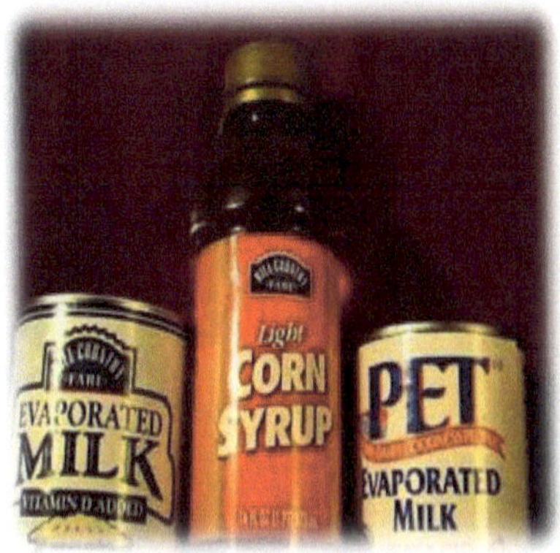

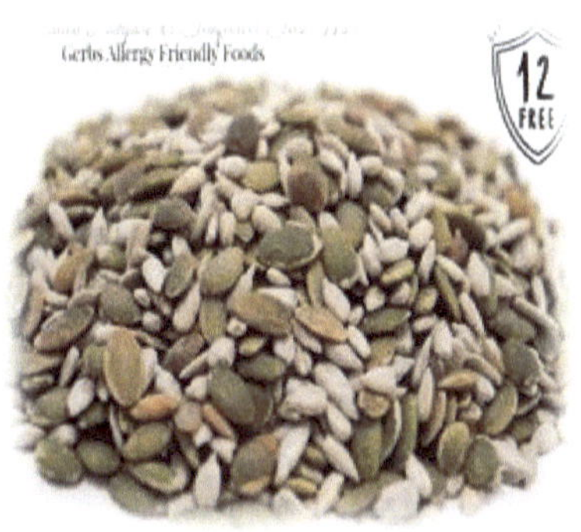

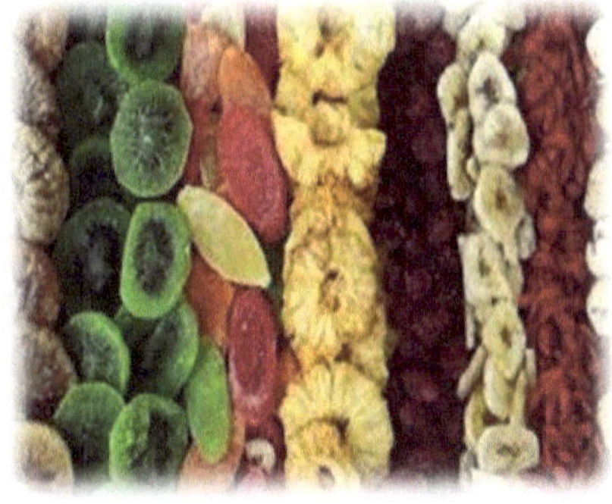

Dried fruits and evaporated and dry milks are also great for storage; they also have a good shelf-like. In addition, Karo-syrup, vitamin C tablets, pumpkin and sunflower seeds are additional food substance that can be stored in your cabinet.

The Benefits of Coffee and Tea

Coffee and tea are great foods to store. They are great beverages to suppress the appetite and help boost the immune system. Coffee is a drink made from coffee beans, a roasted fruit of the "Coffea Arabica" bush. On the other hand, teas are infusion of different types of leaves and seeds. Both foods contain caffeine that stimulate the central nervous system, heart, and muscles. While coffee is higher in both caffeine and antioxidants, you can drink more tea throughout the day to gain equal health benefits.

The Coffee Bean

Coffee is rich in powerful antioxidants, and many people get more antioxidants from coffee than from fruits and veggies combined. It is high in antioxidants and one of the healthiest beverages on the planet. Check out some health benefits:

1. Can Improve Energy Levels
2. Can Help to Burn Fat
3. Can Fight Depression
4. May Lower the Risk to Having a Stroke
5. A Big Source of Antioxidants

Tea Leaves for Storage

1. Peppermint

2. Hibiscus Leaves

3. Spearmint

4. Black Tea

5. Chamomile

6. Green Tea

7. Chai Tea

Avoid Using Tea Bags

Most tea leaves that are in cased in tea bags are likely coated with epichlorohydrin, which is a known carcinogen that is particularly active in hot water. In addition, most tea manufacturers have begun to use plastics like PVC and food-grade nylon as an alternative to the paper tea bags. These teabags introduced to hot water will begin to leach small dose of toxic chemicals that are not good for human consumption. Loose leaf teas are the better buy and healthy and taste better.

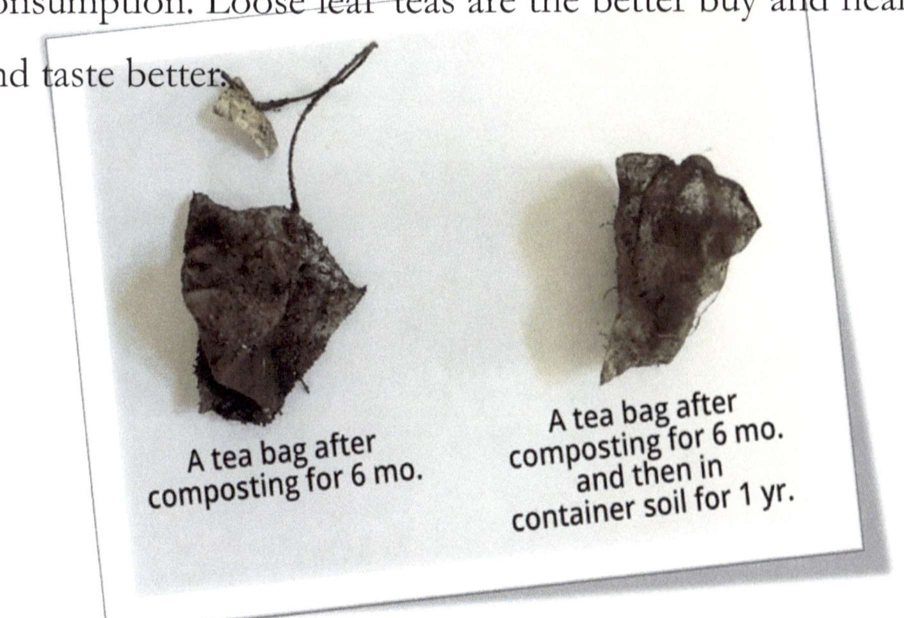

A tea bag after composting for 6 mo.

A tea bag after composting for 6 mo. and then in container soil for 1 yr.

Simple Warm Comforting Tea Beverages

Although coffee is a great diuretic and an appetite suppressant, it can also cause ulcers and stomach pains. Most teas are a great alternative for suppressing the appetite and provides health benefit. It also adds nutritional value when fasting and eating one meal a day, or one meal every other day.

Ginger & Hibiscus Tea

Put the dried hibiscus flowers and ginger, into a measuring cup or pot big enough to hold 8 cups. Cover with the boiling water, and steep for 5 minutes or until you have the desired strength. The longer you leave it to steep, the stronger and more intense the flavor will be. Strain and add honey to taste.

Homemade Chai Tea Recipe

Chai tea is one of my favorite teas; therefore, below is a basic recipe to make and store.

- 12 green cardamom pods
- 1/2 teaspoon whole red peppercorns (optional)
- 1/2 teaspoon whole black peppercorns
- 1 tablespoon fennel seeds
- 1/2 teaspoon coriander seeds
- 1/2 teaspoon whole cloves
- 1 4-inch cinnamon stick
- 3 tablespoons chopped candied ginger
- 1/2 cup loose black tea

Place in a pie tin along with the peppercorns, fennel, coriander, cloves and cinnamon. Toast in the oven for about 5 minutes, or until the spices are fragrant. Remove and cool. Crush spices lightly with a rolling pin or in a mortar and pestle.

Golden Milk or Tea

Golden milk tea is warm and soothing and provides antioxidants. Its great before bedtime, curled up to a good book.

Recipe

- 2 cups of your favorite milk
- 1 tbsp coconut oil
- 1 tsp ginger powder
- 1 tsp cinnamon powder
- ¼ tsp black peppercorn

1 tsp. turmeric powder
Dash of Kosher Salt
Raw Honey to taste
Cinnamon Stick

Instructions

Add turmeric to a saucepan with water and reduce on low to medium-low heat until it begins to form a thick paste. Add in oil, ginger, cinnamon, and salt. Stir until it thickens. Let cool and put in a jar. When ready to use, add a tablespoon to any cup of warm milk that you like. Stir in honey and top it off with a cinnamon stick.

Banana Tea

Bananas are a great source of magnesium & potassium, which help to relax the muscle and regulates the digestive system. It is not only good eaten raw, it makes a delicious tea beverage that can relax the mind, body, and soul.

Banana Tea Recipe

1 banana peel and peel with ends trimmed off

1¼ cup water

1 cinnamon stick

1/4 tsp vanilla extract

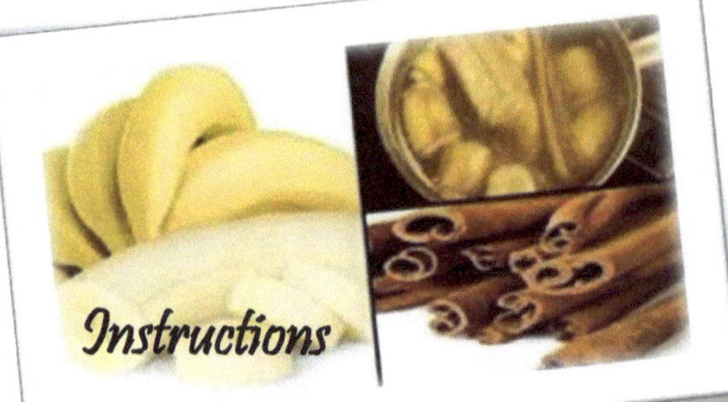

Instructions

Place banana and cinnamon stick in the water and bring to a boil. Cover, reduce heat and simmer on low for 8-10 minutes. Remove from heat and strain out peel. Add vanilla extract (if using) and sweetener if desired before serving. You can also eat the boil banana as well. Just sprinkle cinnamon on top and enjoy!

Drinking A Glass of Warm Water

Drinking a glass of warm water before you start your day can heal the body and aide in digestion. It can also reduce built-up intestinal waste and alleviates gas. There are additional health benefits of drinking a warm glass of water before the start of day such as: bowel regulation, alleviates intestinal pain, sheds excess pounds, improves blood circulation, and slows down the aging process. Drink a glass every morning plain or with a twist of lemon to reap the health benefits and maintaining a healthier life.

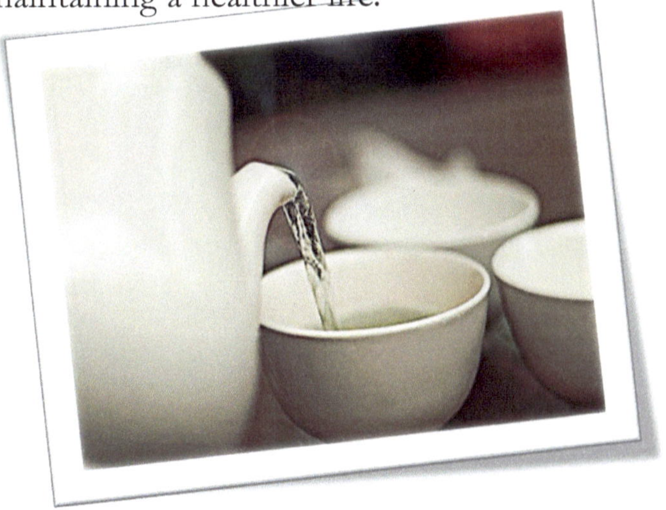

Fermentation & Immune Boosters

Fermenting any citrus fruits and place in a mason jar with raw honey will give your tea and coffee a fruity flavor. Make sure fruits are thinly slice and place inside a mason jar. Fill up the mason jar with raw honey, cover and place in a cool closed cabinet. The juice will infuse with honey and can be used as tea or coffee sweetener. Also, these infused elixirs are great for preventing colds and illnesses.

CAUTION: DO NOT USE STORE BOUGHT HONEY FOR FERMENTATION!

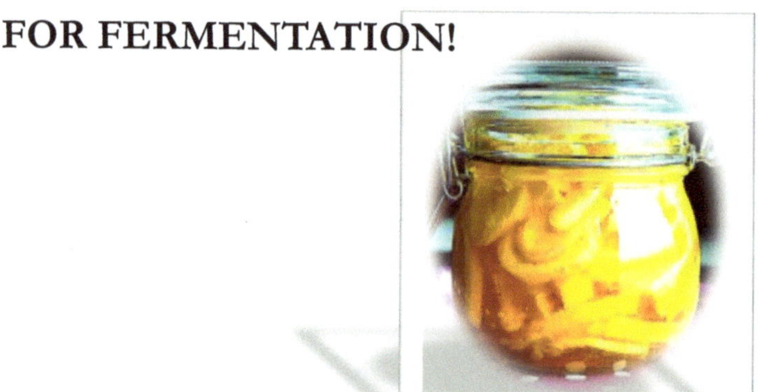

1. Citrus Preserves

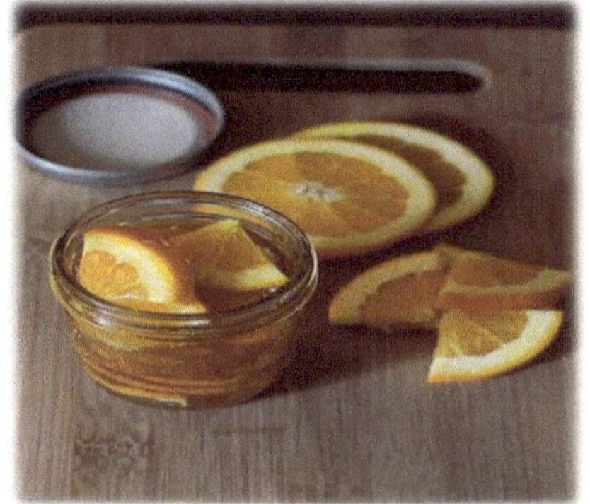

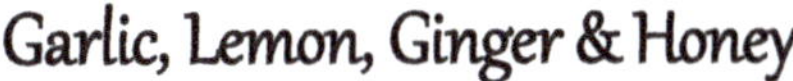
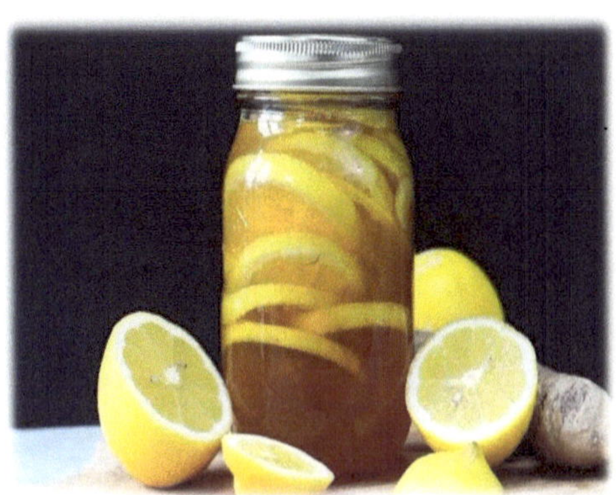

2. Lemon, Garlic, Ginger & Honey

If you ever want to boost your immune system or feel under the weather, these four ingredients will pep you up and bring you comfort.

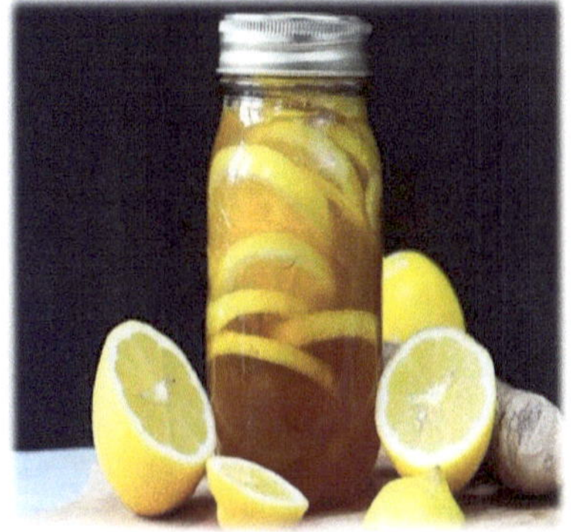

3. Garlic & Honey Fermentation

Garlic and Honey fermentation is great for colds and a boost to your immune system. Place whole garlic cloves in a mason jar with raw honey. Store in a dark cabinet and open the lid every other day to allow the gases to escape for at least a month. Once it becomes a dark liquid it is ready to use.

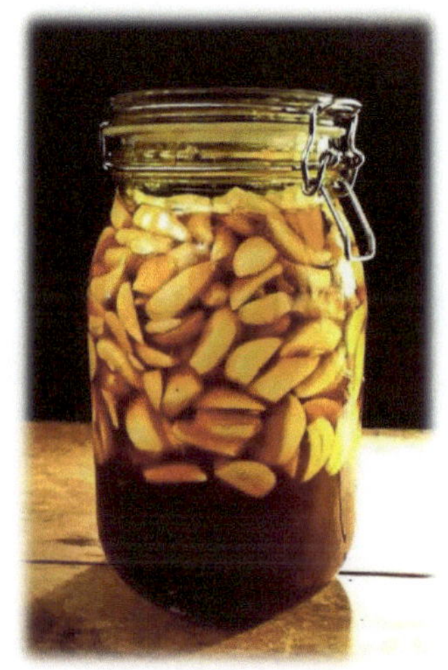

4. Fire Cider Master Tonic Recipe

- 2 to 3 cups raw apple cider vinegar
- ¼ cup garlic minced
- ¼ cup onion minced
- 1/2 cup fresh ginger peeled and grated
- 1/2 cup horseradish peeled and grated
- 2 pieces turmeric root peeled and grated
- 1/4 tsp. cayenne pepper
- 2 minced hot peppers (i.e. jalapeño, habanero)
- 1 Zest and juice from 1 lemon
- 1 Orange thinly sliced
- Raw honey to taste (OPTIONAL)

Combine all the ingredients in a ceramic or glass bowl, except for the vinegar, and honey, and mix well. Transfer the mixture to a one-quart Mason jar. Pour in apple cider vinegar until you fill it to the top. Shake well! Store in a dark, cool place for one month and shake daily. After one month, use cheesecloth or a nut milk bag to strain out the pulp, pouring the vinegar into a clean jar. Be sure to squeeze as much of the liquid as you can from the pulp. You can use the tonic straight or, if you prefer, add 1/4 cup of honey and stir until incorporated to make cider. Taste your cider and add another 1/4 cup of honey until you reach the desired sweetness.

Good Ol'e Fashion Homemade Remedies

Take a teaspoon full of sugar and let the medicine go down!

Back in the days, it was unheard of going to the doctor or the hospital for common illnesses, minor bruises, cuts, or scrapes. In fact, most families did not have health insurance or access to a doctor on a regular basis. Somehow, families managed to stay alive with the help of grandma's old fashion remedies. Today, many old fashion remedies are believed to be outdated and useless. Consequentially, families rely upon pills, over the counter drugs (OTC) that are too expensive and made with chemicals that are toxin and addictive. however, many were cure-alls for almost every ailment. Still today, there's nothing like a bowl of homemade chicken soup especially when you're sick.

19 Old Fashion Remedies and Elixirs

1. Potato Slices on forehead for headaches

2. Olive Oil for eczema

3. Use duct tape for warts

4. Tooth paste for bug bites

5. Beets for Constipation

6. Mix Cumin, Honey, Cinnamon and Ginger for Diarrhea

7. Banana peels for poison ivy

8. Raw honey for acid reflux

9. Blackstrap molasses for constipation

10. Teabags for burns

11. Basil leaves and ginger for fevers

12. A glass of warm milk with a teaspoon of turmeric powder added to it before bed to delineate snoring

13. AN OLD FASHION BABY FORMULA RECIPE
Breast milk is the best!

Breast milk is the best; however, if there is no natural milk around, this recipe will help fill up your baby's stomach. Make sure the liquid vitamin has the code, which stands for Kosher. Once the baby is over 3 months, add weak bean soup without any spices to the formula.

- 2 oz cans evaporated milk

- 32 oz distilled or purified water

- 2 tablespoon Karo-syrup

- 3 Milliliters of poly-vi-sol (liquid vitamins)

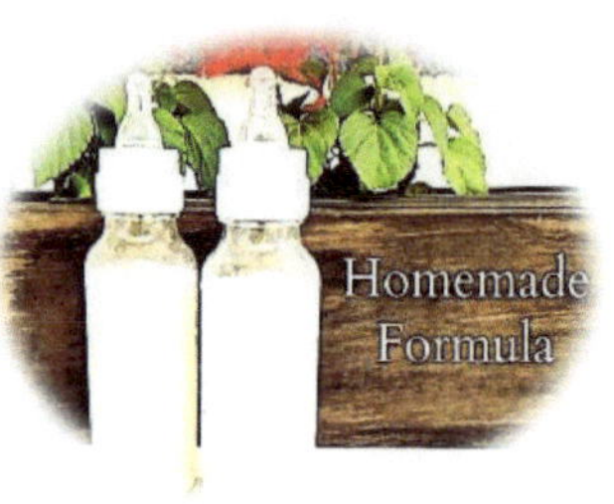

14. Cod Liver Oil

Cod liver oil can naturally help the pain of arthritis. The oil is extracted from cod fish that provides a rich source of EPA and DHA omega-3 fatty acids. According to nutritionists, these are the primary omega-3s you need to support heart health, brain health, eye health, and maternal health.

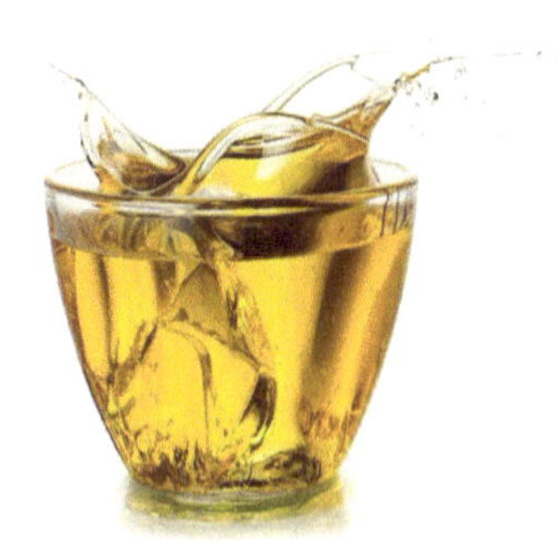

15. Licorice Roots

The licorice root is a plant and aids in healing bad breath; it is an effective agent to fight the bacteria that can cause tooth decay and periodontal disease. The root is used as a dietary aide such as digestive problems, menopausal symptoms, cough, and bacterial and viral infections.

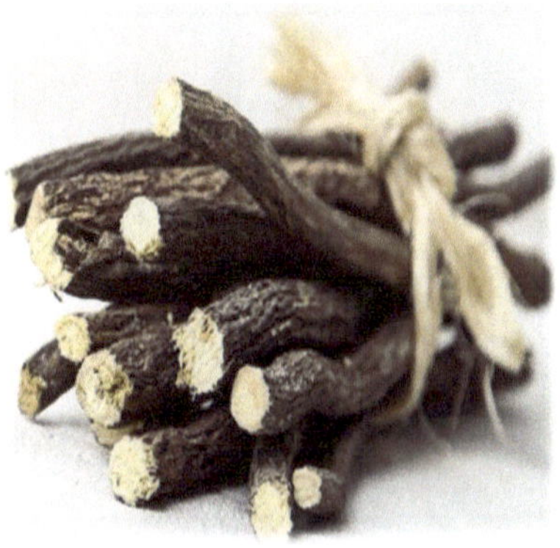

16. Chicory Root

Chicory is a plant; its roots and dried ground parts are used to make medicine. The root is used for high blood pressure, heart failure, loss of appetite, upset stomach, constipation, liver, and gallbladder disorders. It also aids in cancer, and rapid heartbeat. Chicory is a rich source of beta-carotene and the leaves are often eaten like celery.

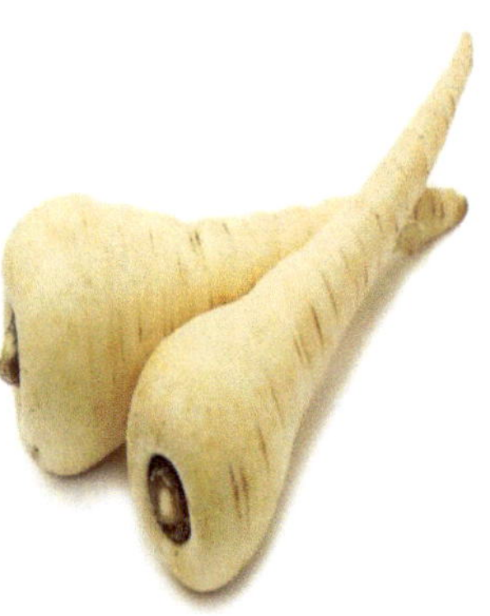

17. Colloidal Silver

Colloidal silver is a mineral, which is used as a dietary supplement and a variety wide range of ailments. The mineral is used for conditions such as infections (i.e. eye and ear infections), cancer, diabetes, arthritis, and much more.

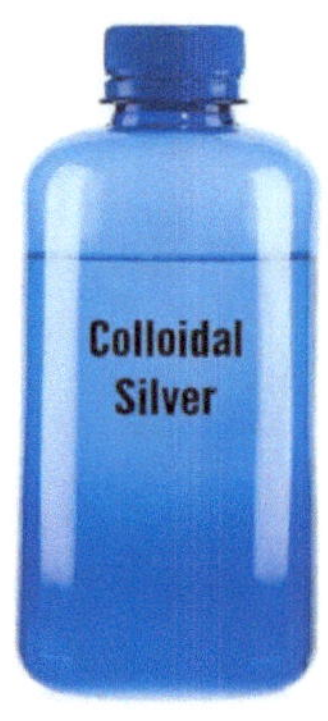

18. Oil of Oregano

Oil of Oregano is a great remedy to fight bacterial and fungal infections. It also boosts immunity from viral infections, and fights off most parasites such as ringworms. Oregano oil has so many healing properties. However, the most common use is for breathing ailments.

1 Cup of Oregano
½ Cup of Olive Oil
Mix well and store in a jar for 2 months. After two months, drain the leaves and place oil in a vial or a glass bottle.

19. Witch Hazel

Witch Hazel is a liquid solution derived from the leaves and bark of a type of shrub that is native to North America. It is an anti-inflammatory agent that helps to relieve the burn of hemorrhoids, applied to the skin and scalp, and soothe sensitive skin. In addition, it can be added to herbal teas and ingested orally in small amounts as a natural treatment to relieve sore throats.

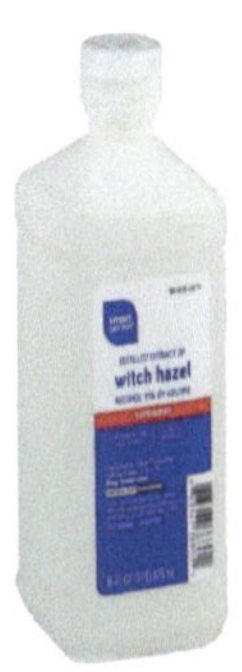

Best Food to Relieve Constipation

1. Dried Prunes
2. Apples (Particularly Granny Smith)
3. Pears
4. Kiwifruit
5. Figs
6. Citrus Fruits
7. Green Vegetables
8. Oatmeal
9. Flaxseed

Green vegetables, fruits and oats are highly rich in insoluble fiber and sugars (i.e. sorbitol, and pectin). In the gut, pectin is rapidly fermented by bacteria to form short-chain fatty acids, which pull water into the colon, softening the stool and decreasing gut transit time.

5 Homeopathic Products that are Harmful to the Body

1. Nu Vomica – Seeds used for rat poison
2. Aconite – A root that contains poisonous chemicals
3. Arnica – Poisonous Plant
4. Cantharis -Lytta Vesicatoria (Spanish Fly or Blister Beetle)
5. Rhus tox – Poison Ivy

Most OTC medication are safe to ingest and will not cause a long-term health risk. Many OTC are labeled homeopathic, but will cause irreputable damage to internal organs. The five homeopathic medicine listed are made from herbs and flowers and insects that are toxic and can cause liver and kidney failure and most likely death. If purchased, only use for atopic purposes such as skin rashes, eczema, and bug bites. **DO NOT INGEST AND RESEARCH INGREDIENTS**!

Conclusion

In this day and time, foods are losing nutritional value and weakening the immune system. My Medicine Cabinet is a basic homeopathic book that provides simple foods, recipes, and home remedies that treat the body and maintain a quality of life. Rather than buy all types of OTC medicines to treat simple illnesses; the recipes and products in this book provides an alternative approach to traditional medicine. In addition, eating the right foods at the right time and storing foods in mason jars will help to maintain a quality of life. Finally, these homeopathic remedies will not only help to boost the immune system, it will also provide information to aide in digestion and avoid fewer visits to the doctor's office.

References

http://www.bisphenol-a.org/human/epoxycan.html

https://www.epicurious.com

https://www.fooducate.com

https://www.greenchildmagazine.com/plastic-in-tea-bags/

https://www.healthline.com/nutrition/best-foods-for-constipation#section2

https://www.myrecipes.com/recipe

https://www.ncbi.nlm.nih.gov/pubmed/19022962

https://nccih.nih.gov/health/licoriceroot

https://www.webmd.com

http://www.whfoods.com

https://yangsnourishingkitchen.com/honey-fermented-garlic/

https://youtu.be/9bupAhuvnb0

Muhammad, Elijah. How to Eat to Live Book 1 and 2.

Personal Note Page

Personal Note Page

Personal Note Page

www.ingramcontent.com/pod-product-compliance
Lightning Source LLC
Chambersburg PA
CBHW040233240726
48664CB00001B/121